Surviving Mold:
No Ego Just Love -

10 Things You Must Do To Get Well Today

Josh Ryan

ISBN: 1514894300
ISBN-13: 978-1514894309

DEDICATION

This is about you. When I was searching, hoping, praying and studying for over 12 years, I had to win. I had to beat biotoxin, C.I.R.S. and mold illness, not only for myself but also so that I could help others as well.

I never gave up fighting and I never gave up hope – nor should you. Make a decision to win and realize that you already have won because God has provided you with the answer – you just have to allow wellness to happen for you too.

This book has an exact step-by-step guide of exactly what I did and what is required for someone to cure or heal themselves from mold exposure and illness. It is my guarantee that there is information in this book that your doctor has never told you and that you haven't read online before.

I will also summarize later in another chapter the hardest hitting, lowest cost, most effective ways to get well by providing a simple and easy to understand plan that requires no thinking, just action.

This book is also dedicated to the people in your life – your family, friends and work relations. Many of these people are not able to understand what you've gone through or continue to go through. This will help them understand why you may be experiencing multiple chemical sensitivities now or mold related issues. These people in your support system need the understanding and compassion to help you create a wellness environment that will extend to all aspects of your life.

Forward

*Warning – common sense and wisdom has been thrown out the window. If you believe that only a doctor can fix you, then that is exactly what will have to happen for you to get well. Always consult with a licensed healthcare practitioner.

It took 12 years of study, trial and error, common sense and logic to solve my challenges. I still have to stay focused on a wellness life and lifestyle to have any energy or athletic ability.

Always remember:

"Results do not equal no results plus a good story or an excuse." – Josh Ryan

Learn to "take yourself lightly but your problem or situation seriously" – My friend and Author C.W. Metcalf

TIME is our most precious treasure because it is LIMITED. We can produce more wealth, but we cannot produce more time. When we give someone our time, we actually give them a portion of our life that we can never take back. Our time is our life.

Isn't it time you got your life back? Isn't it time you started to dream again? It's time to take action now. This is my gift to you, my time writing this and taking over 12 years to study, spending thousands of hours, meeting top doctors and scientists from all over the world and putting everything together.

Make a Decision

I had to make a decision. I had been sick, ill all my life from being exposed to toxic black mold. It stole my energy, attitude, thinking ability, relationships and forced me to surrender.

I've put a plan in place so you don't have to even think, you don't have to read about my story, heartache or experiences – you can skip to the end.

I knew that if I took what I already knew and had learned over 10 years of study, and took massive action with the new information I had discovered, and invested in my health, that I would get better.

I made a decision that I would do everything on my own first before I went to an "expert" in Biotoxin illness and C.I.R.S (Chronic Inflammation Response Syndrome), knowing that it would cost me tens of thousands of dollars I didn't have to go see an expert. Not to mention all of the tests they would want to do to get the numbers they would want to study, all so that they could create a "standardized treatment" and have enough proof for a protocol or funding. I figured I didn't have anything to lose if I took what I already knew, continued to study and then took massive action. I knew that natural therapies and detoxing wouldn't kill me, so I took action.

I discovered some key information that I was missing that made all the difference.

There's a process that anyone must go through in any transformation. Just like the butterfly must come from the cocoon and morph into its beautiful shape, so must you transform into being well and having a wellness life.

I almost quit the things I was doing many times – detox programs, supplements, exercise and other things. Remember that you have control of the gas pedal, brake and steering wheel in your life and you decide how fast you want to go.

Keep in mind that no matter what you do, you're probably going to feel worse before you feel better. Many of the things you will do may cause you to feel like you're having a "herxheimer reaction."

It may seem like you're "peeling layers from an onion" in regards to your road of wellness. However, the reality is you're already healed and well. All you have to do is eliminate the toxins, adapt a wellness lifestyle and take action daily. Stop thinking about stuff that doesn't serve or support your wellness; it doesn't matter, and it's a waste of time and energy.

I almost even quit from writing this book, but you deserve to save yourself from years of torment. Get well today. I just want to make a difference.

Waking Up

Imagine being born today at your current age with all of your life experiences, wounds, injuries, love, friendships, success and failure only to realize you have been sick your entire life.

You've had low energy, vision problems, flu-like symptoms, sinus problems, and plugged and swollen lymph nodes. I thought this was how life was for other people and that everyone had a similar experience as me. It's all I had known.

My tongue was white from the mold that had grown on it; my tonsils were swollen and full of stones and bacteria, and my neck was also swollen. It always felt like I was going to swallow the roof of my mouth.

It's like you've been driving your car down the road in a heavy fog, but this fog was real and literal and affected your vision every day. It made it hard to see, focus, read and think clearly.

Up until recently, that's what my story has been. I don't have a gauge or anything to compare life to before mold and Biotoxin illness.

I am very grateful to be out of the fog and disease now. It's been a long, hard road. It's cost me a lot of time, energy, emotion, relationships, income, and more.

I've always wanted to make a difference in a big way in the lives of people and the life of a special lady. Not for my own gain, but just to have the ability to give value to people and share my experience and knowledge so that others don't have to suffer for 30 years or even 1 more year.

I know that many people have ended their own lives or thought about it because they think there's no hope or that a doctor can't fix them. All it takes is some new education and understanding and the belief that all problems and challenges have already been solved but one must learn to "take themselves lightly but their problem or situation seriously." In other words, stay focused on your outcome with faith, create a vision and read and focus on it day and night with plenty of positive emotions. I promise you that God and the Universe will deliver. They have to. It's written in Universal law, and that's how things work for everyone everywhere.

If you don't believe it, start to read or listen to audio versions of books such as *Biology of Belief*, *Think and Grow Rich*, *The Magic of Believing*, and *As a Man Thinketh*, or read Gregg Braden's work. Many of these you can even listen to for free on youtube.com.

**Before you read this book, please make a commitment to leave a review of this book on amazon.com so we can help more people. Remember there are other people just like you and I that are fighting a battle from toxic mold. I put this information together to accelerate healing and wellness.

How Do You Know If You or Someone You Know Is

Sick?

Researchers believe that about 25% of people have a genetic inheritance that makes them unable to eliminate mold toxins. For some reason, the body doesn't recognize these invaders and doesn't eliminate them. What happens is that all of the stuff from your lymph system goes to your liver and the bile made from the liver gets recirculated through your body. Thus, your body is constantly living in a garbage dump. Imagine what would happen if your glass was almost full of water and then you added more – it overflows. This is why it's so important to change your lifestyle by eliminating alcohol, gluten and other things. Your "cup" is probably already full, so don't add to it. Instead let's help your liver by doing special detoxes and other healthy things for it.

It's believed that 25 million Americans have some degree of a mold toxin illness, though it is called MS, Parkinson's, chronic fatigue, fibromyalgia, rheumatoid arthritis, cancer and ADD/ADHD. This is why it's key to learn and study about this illness on your own while living a lifestyle that is in accordance with how you were designed to operate. There is a lot of research showing that most cases of ADD are actually due to mold exposure. Kids or people aren't able to think clearly, see or sit still – sound familiar?

Mold toxins attach to fat cells, and they continue to release inflammation. The result is chronic inflammation with symptoms such as fatigue, pain, brain fog, out of control weight gain and loss of sex drive. When someone has the flu, their symptoms are not caused directly by the viruses. The symptoms are caused by the resulting inflammatory response produced by the immune system. Mold toxins can cause symptoms similar to a permanent case of the flu.

In my experience, it felt like I had the flu every day; I ached, had no energy, couldn't think clearly, had a hard time seeing and a difficult time reading, especially computer screens.

The result of this increasing inflammation can be severe pain, blood sugar problems, nerve damage, reduced circulation, autoimmune diseases, cancer and symptoms that resemble advanced heart disease.

This also affects your athletic ability as the tissues of the body don't receive enough oxygen. This is why supporting your cardiovascular health is key – more on this later.

After I would try to really have a decent workout, I could have a crash that lasted for days. Doing certain exercises and limiting others is important. This inflammation can even result in gluten intolerance! There is tons of data that prove humans should not be eating any gluten period. It creates inflammation and disease in the body even for "healthy people." You also can check out wheatbellyblog.com and other sites related to gluten for more information.

Keep in mind that air quality tests are not always accurate. If you smell mold or musty smells, you probably have a problem.

One of the grossest things I remember is that when I would wake up each day and throughout my day, my tongue was coated with a white substance. I would scrape and scrape it, and it would all come right back.

Another issue I struggled with recently was a clogged lymphatic system, especially in my neck. The lymph system doesn't have a pump like the heart so doing things like "rebounding" or alternating hot and cold water in the shower is important. The biggest impact came from Mullein and lobelia herb in a paste that I rubbed on my neck. This finally forced whatever junk was stuck in my neck and tonsils to go away. It always felt like I was going to swallow the roof of my mouth and tonsils because they were backfilled with so much poison. There are many videos you can watch online for free to learn about massages you can do to manually pump your lymphatic system and drain it.

Other symptoms may include: fatigue, weakness, muscle cramps, light sensitivity, mood swings, white tongue, chronic sinus and tonsil stones, night sweats, excessive urination, static shocks, focus/concentration, excessive thirst and many others.

One of the key indicators of a Biotoxin illness is your vision. Oftentimes the optic nerve in the eye is not getting enough blood flow. On his survivingmold.com website, Dr. Shoemaker has a VCS test or Visual Contrast Sensitivity test that evaluates how well you can see contrast. With 96% accuracy, they believe if you fail this test there may be a Biotoxin in your body.

For more information from Dr. Loyd, visit www.royalrife.com/mold_toxins.pdf

Keep in mind there is an information war going on. This psychological warfare is being perpetuated by lobbyists who put money into the pockets of people in power at the FDA, School Systems, Politicians and many others. Follow the money and profits and you'll discover the truths. You must discover truths for you and ask yourself, "How did God design my body to operate?" What are the things I should be doing on a daily basis and what should I be putting into it?

Multiple Chemical Sensitivity

You may not be aware that you're experiencing some sort of MCS. Multiple Chemical Sensitivity is a term used for people who are sensitive to chemicals, perfumes and other odors. Some "experts" believe that people are making it up in their heads.

The symptoms are flu-like – dizziness, fatigue, headaches, gastrointestinal tract issues, inflammation and others.

Some believe it's the odors of these chemicals that give people a knee-jerk reaction to feel sick. This could make logical sense as I know that mold smells instantly make my body repulse.

If someone wears or sprays perfume, cologne, or hairspray around me, it wipes me out and I get really frustrated. Regardless, let's not forget that perfumes are, in fact, TOXIC and chemicals. Why would you want them on your body even if you don't experience MCS symptoms?

Stop using chemicals and being in environments that have chemicals, and encourage others around you to support your life and lifestyle.

Ear Infections and Your Lymphatic System

I remember the first time I saw an ear, nose and throat doctor (ENT). I had an ear infection which had to have been in there for at least 6 months. My ears were plugged; it felt like I was going to swallow the roof of my mouth. My throat and lymph nodes in my neck were swollen. Every day I would pull huge white chunks out of my tonsils.

The doctor vacuumed out my ears and had a look inside them. He asked if I had had a lot of ear infections in my life. I said not that I know of. He told me I had so much scarring on my ear drums that I must have had chronic ear infections all of my life.

That was pretty interesting to hear after all these years not only of not being able to see clearly through my eyes but also not being able to hear through healthy ears as well. I never thought there was anything wrong with my hearing, but I can only imagine where I would be or what I would be like had I been able to think, see and hear clearly like a healthy person.

It also always felt like I had something stuck in the space between my ear and my neck in the Eustachian Tube. This was probably due to the major blockage in my lymphatic system in my neck, tonsils and sinus.

Even after I felt better from all of the detoxes and supplements and was almost feeling "normal," even though I had no real concept of what "normal" is as I've felt ill all my life, I still had blockage in my neck and tonsils. Plus I had massive tonsil stones that would come out each day, and it felt like I was going to swallow the roof of my mouth. I went back into some of the things I had studied and read, particularly Dr. Christopher's work. He mentions that Mullein and Lobelia herbs can be taken as a tea and also rubbed on the skin to force the stuff out of the lymphatic system.

After years of my neck being plugged and massive tonsil stones coming out daily, for a few days I used a large quantity of his Glandular System paste and rubbed it all over my neck. It worked!

Dr. Christopher also has a Glandular System herbal supplement that you can take internally. I have used both of them at the same time for major results.

Also, buy a rebounder – you know, a mini trampoline. Studies show that jumping on a trampoline will help flush out your lymph system.

Alternate hot water and cold water a minute at a time, back and forth during your shower, but always make sure to end on cold.

Learn lymphatic massages or have a partner do them with you.

Dr. Christopher also says for inflamed tonsils, salivary glands, and neighboring lymph glands to keep garlic in the mouth constantly during the morning and throughout the day. Put a new piece of garlic in your mouth at mid to late day. The garlic absorbs the poisons, so be sure not to eat it.

Dr. Christopher was one of the foremost experts and pioneers in herbal and alternative medicine. Dr. Schultz of Herbdoc.com was a student of Dr. Christopher and has created some amazing products.

Make your life easy by thinking in terms of simple solutions. Stop complicating things and just take action. Know that your healing and wellness lifestyle already exists and step into it. Buy a copy of Think and Grow Rich, master chapter 2 on burning desire and chapter 4 on autosuggestion. Go on Youtube and listen to Claude Bristol and the Magic of Believing.

Injuries and Accidents

I don't want to go into too many details, but there is a lot of research and information showing that people who have been in car accidents or who have had other traumas commonly experience C.I.R.S. These people experience the same symptoms of chronic inflammation as those who have been exposed to Biotoxins. This is a great article and a good starting point for more information.

http://articles.mercola.com/sites/articles/archive/2012/07/22/mold-and-other-chronic-diseases.aspx

There are many white labeled products with hyaluronic acid, BioCell Collagen and Collagen type 2. If you have a back injury, joint injury or soft tissue damage you should be on a product with these ingredients.

BioCell Collagen is a trademarked name and licensed to many different products. There is a tremendous amount of science and research behind it. Try it for yourself it works and is very inexpensive.

Alcohol

The good news is you're going to stop drinking alcohol altogether. The other good news is you're going to stop drinking alcohol. Don't forget that alcohol is toxic; oftentimes it is full of gluten and other toxins that are harmful to the body.

Make your liver your friend and not your enemy. Your liver needs all the love and support it can get from you. Your lymph system is dumping all its garbage into your liver, and your liver is probably dealing with circulating toxic bile.

Dealing With Family Members and Friends – What They Need to Understand

Listen, if you're a friend or family member of a person that's been affected by a Biotoxin illness like mold, Lyme or any other disease, there are a few things to understand. You may live in the same home and not think you're sick, or you may not have any health challenges yourself. That doesn't mean it's not very real to the person with this book, or your friend or family member who is ill.

My parents had a mold-filled house, though I never had it confirmed officially. I could smell it, I saw it in the attic, and black mold coated the dirty laundry towel hamper. Not to mention I had every symptom, failed every mold type test I had ever taken and was very sick. My parents and siblings didn't appear to have the same health challenges as me, though looking back I can almost guarantee that my sister's major allergies to gluten, my parent's health issues and my other sister's thyroid and hormone issues are in direct relation.

Sometimes people thought I was just making stuff up. The lack of respect and ignorance from family members can be frustrating and can make you feel like you want to end any relationship with them altogether.

You need to do everything to get the problem solved first or move to a new home. Make it your number one goal and focus to get out of there now and get your loved one to safety. If that's not an option, get your loved one to safety without you. Get them on a detox program and take the actions that I took to get well.

Your loved one deserves to be healthy; after all you love them and care about them, right?

Detox

Let's get the poisons out of your body. One of the best ways is a product called CholestePure by Pure Encapsulations. For some reason, it binds to the mold toxins and helps you get them out of your system. Taking this product may make you feel worse before you feel better, so start slow.

I was so broke financially and so tired and exhausted and stressed out, but I decided to spend the $500 to buy Dr. Schultz's "incurables program" from herbdoc.com. Looking back, I feel like there were a couple components I could have done without, but this program is amazing. You start off with his intestinal cleanse and liver cleanse in week number one, combined with tea and juicing every day. Week two you do his kidney cleanse and then alternate back to week one for 30 days. Dr. Schultz has helped many people learn how to use the power of foods and herbs to heal themselves. Besides, it can't hurt – these are the nutrients that you're supposed to be putting in your body anyway!

If you do nothing else, do his intestinal cleanse and liver cleanse along with picking up a copy of his book or ask for a free PDF version of "There Are No Incurable Diseases." You need to help your liver cleanse itself and get really healthy. Your liver is a major key to your healing, so become a nondrinker and stop putting poisons in your body. It is thought that it takes 6 months for the liver to regenerate itself, so keep this in mind.

There are no excuses in life – only results, and results do not equal no results plus a good story or an excuse.

Liquid zeolite has shown significant results in pulling out heavy metals and toxins in the body as well. Do your research on liquid zeolite and see if it makes sense for you.

Chlorophyll is an inexpensive green liquid that will also help you in making more alkaline while detoxing the body as well. This also works great with juicing.

Cream of tartar is known to help eliminate candida and mold in the body. Of all the research I've done, I found that Dr. Wong's Candessence product is extremely potent. It also has a few other ingredients that may help in mold detox.

Diatomaceous Earth is another low-cost product that is great to have on hand. The only one worth buying is food grade from a company called Permaguard. DE is known to help "cut up" and kill parasites while pulling out heavy metals and toxins from the body.

Diet

It's time for you to eat and drink for how the body was designed. There are things you need to let go of such as alcohol, coffee, gluten, and most things that grow under the ground. Many foods like coffee are moldy or have Mycotoxins. It really is simple – stop drinking it and ingesting other known mold-filled foods and see how you feel.

I'm going to help you use common sense and logic. You need to test how foods make you feel. Nuts and grains are harvested and then sit in silos and develop mold. Who knows how long they sit in these silos? Also think about the toxic chemicals that are typically used on conventional crops today.

It's also a good idea to learn to identify foods that have gluten as it is not good for anyone. It causes inflammation, leaky gut and other diseases. Not to mention that it creates mucus in the body.

I'm not a fan of dairy anymore either. Many researchers believe the adverse effects to dairy are not caused by lactose but by a protein called A1. Over 90% of cows have and produce this A1 protein. There are other dairy alternatives out there that are from A2 producing cows. Learn more about this if you're still eating dairy. For thousands of years, dairy (from A2 cows) has been one of the greatest nutrients ever and is known to cause healing. Keep in mind that dairy causes mucus.

Some believe the "Mucus-less Diet" is the way to go. Use common sense and eat grass fed meats and organic vegetables. Better yet, juice for at least 30 days and see how you feel.

Garlic is a great addition to your diet. It has over 33 sulfur compounds. Sulfur helps fight fatigue. Sulfur also plays an important role in energy, proper insulin function, detoxing and more.

Sometimes I'll eat something I shouldn't like sugary foods or drinks, gluten or other things. I notice that sometimes it totally wipes me out. I end up taking charcoal/bentonite clay and also the CholestePure product to help pull those toxins out. Typically I get back to normal very quickly.

People who have been exposed to mold make antibodies to gliadin, which is a protein found in wheat. This is what causes the inability to tolerate gluten grains. A diet high in sugar and starches causes the insulin to spike, which makes things worse.

Research has shown that leptin resistance is a major issue in hormones and weight loss. When these leptin receptor sites are blocked, levels rise. The leptin packs into fat cells until the toxins are removed. This is why people with high leptin levels can gain weight even with low calorie intake.

This leptin receptor blockage creates a blockage of a hormone called MSH. When MSH is low, melatonin production will be low too, which results in sleep problems.

The obvious thing here is you can take things like melatonin, valerian root or other natural sleep aids.

Another thing that is great is "Earthing." Humans used to walk the earth barefoot and were constantly connected to the earth's energy. Studies show that by being connected to the earth's energy you actually throw off negatively charged dirty energy and recharge your body in a positive way. You can do your own research on Earthing and even buy Earthing bed sheets that have many silver strands running through the fitted bed sheet. The sheet is then plugged into the ground outlet of the 3 prong outlet in your wall. At some point, that ground wire is connected to the earth, thus you are connected to the earth.

I think a lot of people don't realize that they have a lot of food allergies, especially from Dairy. Try a mucusless diet regime.

Exercise

I know it may be hard or very tiring to exercise. Get yourself a rebounder and jump on it daily to flush the lymphatic system. Also get one hour of exercise in every day. Take it slow and go easy on yourself. Treat yourself nicely and don't get upset that you can't do things you once could do before.

It's a good idea to get your body fat down. You don't have to be an Adonis, remember that toxins store in fat. It may be hard for you to work out or you may crash for days after a workout. Take it easy and go slow. Make sure you're consistent and exercise daily.

Get out there and move! You MUST exercise for at least 1 hour per day. Read Dr. Schultz' book "There Are No Incurable Diseases."

Taking Action & What To Take

Let's use "common sense" and a logical approach to getting well.

If you're like me, you've probably tried almost everything or maybe you think you have. I studied for over 12 years searching and praying for answers, learning how the body works on a cellular level and what things do. I have invested hundreds and thousands of hours into studying wellness.

I have met and spoke with the President Emeritus of the Naturopathic Society several times, as well as heads of Naturopathic universities, Johns Hopkins, DFW, top research scientists, the former head of the United States Patent and Trademark Office for new discoveries in health, and the list goes on.

I am going to keep everything very simple. If you'd like to do research and study all of the hard core science, go right ahead. Alternatively, you could just focus on the results and getting well by letting me help guide you to the success God has given to you and is waiting for you to claim.

Part of it is you have to have faith that your creator designed you perfectly and that your body is programmed and designed to heal itself, which it is.

Science is now showing that it's not genetics that's the problem. Meaning even if you're one of the "25% that doesn't expel mold toxins well", it doesn't mean that there's something wrong with you. The real issue is inflammation and toxins and other things interfering with the communication system of your body.

This means that if you fix the communication system, your body will, in fact, heal and return to a place of wellness. Read this page again. Your body will heal itself – yes you.

Furthermore, if you listen to Dr. Bruce Lipton in the *Biology of Belief,* he goes into another form of science through thought and emotion that operates on a higher level above the issues and disease on the cellular level that, in fact, controls everything.

Most people believe they have to go to a doctor to get well. If that's your belief, then this is not for you. I believed that my creator made me perfect and whole, even if there was a "genetic issue" of me not being able to deal with expelling Biotoxins. As I know from my study, research and meeting with top experts from around the world, Science has now proven that it's not the genes that are the issue. It's the operating system above the genes that controls if you're well or not.

More specifically, God didn't make crap on the DNA level. You are already healthy and perfect. You may be experiencing a polluted and toxic environment inside your body, and on the cellular level that perfect message is not being expressed perfectly because of all of the poisons, toxins and things interfering with your communication system.

This is exciting news!!! Rejoice, because you're already perfect and equipped with everything you need for your wellness and healing, and nothing is wrong with you.

Trauma and Spiritual Wounds

We're all wounded people. I remember seeing a T-Shirt that read: "Be Kind To Everyone For They Are Fighting A Battle Too." Shit happens in life – loss of loved ones, illness, loss of income or a job, relational problems, car accidents and other trauma happens in life. I believe that those things actually wound your soul.

One of my mentors would say that humans have a negative imprinted memory and it does have a physical weight, though small, that attaches to the soul. Another one of my mentors would say that these negative engrams create a charge in the body which further attracts other emotional events and things into your life.

If you're a Christian, you may believe that soul wounds are real and do in fact happen, including generational soul wounds that are passed down. The Bible calls these iniquities. My favorite ministry is Katie Souza based out of Phoenix, Arizona. Her main focus is helping people eliminate these soul wounds through very specific prayers and Biblical Scriptures. I highly recommend her programs such as "Banking in the Glory," "Live Free and Escape the Trap of Bitterness," "Made Perfect in Weakness" and many others. Bitterness causes major torment inside of you and your life and will bring a curse of the curse to ALL aspects of your life. Dig into her ministry and teachings from Scripture and you'll see that many disease states are caused by bitterness, which can cause additional states of illness and problems as well.

You can learn more about her ministry at www.katiesouza.com.

I worked with a best-selling author that worked with people who experience difficulty, trauma and change in life; he wanted to discover why two people could have the same experience in life and yet be totally different. Many would be bitter and others would create incredible states of mind and attitudes despite their circumstances.

Most people don't pray properly, regardless of faith. Jesus' translation of "ask and you shall receive" has been perverted through translation. According to Gregg Braden and the Lost Scrolls of the Dead Sea, the original translation was: "Ask without hidden motive, be surrounded by your answer, be enveloped by what you desire that your gladness be full. So far you have not done this and prayers have gone unanswered." In other words, whatever it is that you want, see it as done, and give thanks that it is already done. The key is to first bring in God's glory through a massive amount of energy movement with your emotions through gratitude. Oftentimes music will help in bringing this creative power and light inside of you.

Glyconutrients

Most people are not aware that since 1994 there have been 4 Nobel Prizes in medicine for studying and theorizing this communication system. Every cell in the human body is coated with millions of what are called Glycoform structures. These structures are made from a protein and many specific Glyconutrients. There are over 10 known Glyconutrients that coat cell surfaces.

Your body continuously makes them, otherwise you'd be dead. However, being that you probably don't eat the foods that are dense and rich with these nutrients, why not supplement them? To create each one of these key nutrients, your body has to do several enzymatic processes to produce just one of these key compounds. This is a very taxing process on the body and nutrients, and nutrition must be in place for an ample amount for wellness to take place.

Studies have shown that these nutrients also help recognize and control the inflammatory molecules and that they are literally are the alphabet or communication system of the human body. These molecules are the very thing that expresses your DNA throughout the rest of your body. Think about what would happen if you removed the vowels from this sentence: t w l d b h rd t r d r ght? It would be hard to read, right?

A well-known, very famous musician's home in New Orleans was flooded from a hurricane. He got sick and found out that he was poisoned from mold and biotoxins. Someone educated him about Glyconutrients and he decided to take mass quantities. He was able to quickly overcome his biotoxin illness.

The company I am speaking of that makes these Glyonutrients is called Mannatech out of Texas. I have no affiliation with them. However, their products are life changing. Due to a lawsuit and our government being controlled by the drug industry, Mannatech is no longer publishing scientific data to the public. I can tell you based on the doctors, scientists and my own research of over 10 years of studying their technology, that it is real and it is sound.

On another note, I have seen the studies on these nutrients and how they help the body produce its own stem cells. Spending money on spinal cord or embryonic stem cells seems inferior, and the costs are out of this world. It makes no sense to have stem cells generated in a lab when your own body can produce far more stem cells with the right nutrients. I still have the videos from the presentation done before the Senate that show these facts.

They also have a product called Immunostart that has lactoferrin and bovine colostrum. Colostrum is what comes out of the breast or teat first for the newborn to get a jump start with their immune system. These compounds have also been shown to help detox and pull heavy metals out of the body.

The key in glycoscience that you need to know is that these nutrients are found in mother's breast milk; that's how safe they are. They determine which blood type you are; that's how important they are. They coat every cell surface in the human body. It is how the good guys communicate and eliminate waste, how the immune system determines friend from foe and how information is transferred.

I have many of the studies, research papers, and videos from top scientists and doctors from all over the world on this subject.

Please understand and keep in mind that drugs of the future are based on this science. Why? It's simple – drug companies believe that by attaching, programming or tagging their drug to specific glycoform shapes or combinations that they can target specific cells inside the body. That's great and everything, but why not instead get what God intended for you to have from nature and avoid the problems all together?

Enzymes

Systemic enzymes were discovered by the Germans over 50 years ago. These enzymes play a key role in inflammation and eating away fibrin in the body. Basically, the number of these enzymes decreases as you age and after you hit age 27, you have a limited supply available. This is why children are able to heal so quickly because these enzymes are in abundance in the body.

They're known to clean the blood, eat fibrin/scar tissue, and fight viruses and bacteria while also being immune system modulators. Keep in mind that fibrin and scar tissue is building up in virtually all parts of your body.

I had a muscle in my upper back area that was cramped for 15 years from a car accident. Nothing I did helped, until a few days on these powerful enzymes. It was like the muscle finally relaxed.

From this same car accident, my lower back was damaged with a disc pushed into my spinal canal. These enzymes, glyconutrients and a few other things have brought me to the point of functioning like a normal, healthy, athletic man – able to play all sports and do everything pain free.

Please do your own research on systemic enzymes. I tried several products, probably almost every one of them available on the market. I found that Dr. William Wong and his product Zymessence was by far the best. Though it does cost a little more than others, it is far more effective and you don't have to take as much. I won't go a day without them. The thing that sets Dr. Wong's Zymessence apart from other enzyme products is he figured out how to enteric coat the individual enzymes inside the capsule. What this means is they're not killed by your stomach acid and thus have a much higher efficacy than other products on the market that only coat the outside of the pill. Take my word and experience for it. It's by far the best product I've tried.

People with Cystic Fibrosis have fibrin that builds up in the lungs, and thus they're not able to breathe properly. Most people with CF don't live past their 20's because they don't have much of any enzyme production to speak of. I have had a couple of close personal friends with CF. One, in fact, has taken action with many of these supplements and lifestyle adjustments for wellness. He is very healthy, especially for someone with CF, and is now 40 years old.

These enzymes are also awesome to have on hand after a workout or after experiencing knee, ankle or sports related injuries. If athletes loaded up on these enzymes, they would see how much quicker the healing process can be and how much better they would feel.

Keep in mind that mold exposure, Lyme's Disease and other Biotoxin illnesses are being thrown into one umbrella in the medical field called C.I.R.S or Chronic Inflammation Response Syndrome. That's great! This means if you can eliminate the poisons and toxins from your body while getting the inflammation down, you WILL FEEL GOOD!

Start slow, but you can take several capsules per day. People who are on blood thinners should consult their doctor. I am not aware of any LD50, meaning these enzymes do not have a lethal dose and won't kill you. Like all food and natural products, they are just that – food. If it's safe for you to eat that hamburger and all the other stuff you eat; I'm sure taking any of the products I took or continue to take is fine.

Iodine

Help your body and thyroid out by getting an iodine supplement. Even just a simple 2% Lugol's solution will do. What I often do is put several drops on the inner side of my arms and then I rub them together. Almost all humans are lacking iodine, and this key ingredient will assist your body in making hormones. You will probably notice instant energy from using iodine, and the best part is it's very inexpensive.

Probiotics

There is massive data that shows eating fermented foods like kimchi and sauerkraut is the best way to get healthy bacteria into the gut. However, for people who have been exposed to biotoxins, it might not be the best thing for you. Test it and see how you feel.

There's a small company out of Idaho called Living Streams Mission. These guys make the strongest and most potent probiotic I've ever taken. When you read the direction, they say only start with one drop of their liquid probiotics and to start by taking it through the skin. Let me tell you, they are not kidding. This stuff is extremely powerful. http://www.livingstreamsmission.com/

Dr. Mercola from www.mercola.com also offers some quality probiotics in a pill form. These are the ones I currently prefer to take.

Rob Keller MD Glutathione

There are many glutathione products on the market. Glutathione is the main antioxidants that your body produces with the right nutrients. Glutathione is known to help detox the body and also for increasing energy production.

If you decide to use glutathione, buy the original Rob Keller MD glutathione product. There are many others on the market that claim to have science and a Multi-Level Marketing MAX INTL that sell theirs for two to three times the price. I have tried them all, and the original Rob Keller MD formula is the best by far and the most affordable.

The bottom line is Rob Keller is the foremost expert in Glutathione and Glutathione research. www.robkellermd.com

Studies show that non pasteurized whey protein will in fact increase Glutathione in the body. In my experience, it is a good idea to eliminate mucus-causing foods such as dairy, eggs, breads, pastas, gluten and others. These create inflammation and cause diseases.

Astaxanthin

Astaxanthin (pronounced asta-zanthin) has been discovered as one of the most powerful antioxidants yet.

It can help you recover from workouts faster, increase your strength, and reduce joint and muscle soreness.

Look up Astaxanthin and what it does for eyesight. This is why I began taking Astaxanthin because of my brain fog and vision fog. It does help and is a great product to have.

I buy my Astaxanthin from Dr. Mercola, but recently I saw it at Costco. I have not tried the Costco brand yet. See Mercola.com.

Sinus Health

If you're like me, then you have probably struggled with your sinus health. I had nose bleeds for over 6 months when I first moved back into that house. Then I bought a Hepa Filter with UV and my nose stopped bleeding, but that didn't help the swelling in my sinus, tonsils and neck.

I was turned on to a natural product called Sino Fresh. Sino Fresh is a nasal spray with essential oils that are known to kill mold. It works – try it for yourself. It's a lot better than constantly shooting drugs up into your nose.

It is believed that many people who have been exposed to mold have staph living in their sinuses and that they won't get better until this staph and bacteria are removed.

B Vitamins

Keep in mind that nerve gas is made from mold, so helping the nerves with things like vitamins B is a good thing to help open up the pathways for the nerves. From the research I've read and my own experimenting, B6 with P5P, as well as Niacin, are great B vitamins to have.

The best way to get any nutrients is from FOOD; however, sometimes trial and error on your own is a good thing.

Clean Air

There is plenty of research that shows Thieves Oil diffused into the air will kill viruses, bacteria and mold. There are a couple of multi-level companies, Young Living and Doterra, that have Thieves Oil. They both seem to be high quality; however, it comes with the expense. I recently found an inexpensive version on amazon.com, but I don't have enough experience with it to say if it's as good or not. I would stick with high quality essential oils. The inferior ones could be toxic to you and your health.

Let me make something clear. All cars today, whether new or old, have mold in them. Most people rarely or never change their cabin air filters either. I bought an essential oil diffuser that plugs into the power outlet. I have read many stories where people were sick because they were breathing in the toxins in their car and not at home. Just remember that all cars are moldy.

Clearing The Lungs

One of the things I immediately did was bought a nebulizer. I also got myself a large bottle of silver solution from silverlungs.com.

You simply take distilled water and distilled water only with the silver solution and breathe in. I can't say for sure how much this helps, though getting the silver in through the lungs is one of the fastest ways and plus you get the benefit of helping the lungs clear out and heal.

Breathe again – do breathing exercises. If you don't know what to do, go on YouTube and see what people are doing to get their oxygen levels up.

I see deals all the time online from Amazon Local, Groupon, Living Social and others for HBOT. Hyperbaric Oxygen Therapy is awesome and will help heal the body very quickly. Do your research on it and try it for yourself.

There are many herbs that can and will help clear the lungs such as lobelia and others. Do your own research on known herbs that will help clean and clear the lungs.

Mindset

Winning the mind game by focusing on the results that you want to have and not on the problems or challenges is what's going to move you forward.

Listening to things like *Biology of Belief* or some of Gregg Braden's work may help. Really make a plan and a decision and write it on paper – read it morning and night. Not just your health and wellness goals but all of your goals. Spend at least 30 minutes at night or while you're lying in bed giving thanks for all of the things you want as if they have already happened.

Learn to overcome ALL bitterness. This is key if you want to be well and live a wellness life. This includes bitterness towards other groups of people, events in your live, events in the past, your circumstances or any other bitterness you may have.

Best Money Spent & Protocol

You should always consult with your Health Care Provider. I accept no responsibility for you using common sense and logic. Keep in mind this is what I personally did and what works for me. I happen to be a human, so maybe it'll work for you too.

If you're on a limited budget, the best things to do and buy are:

CholestePure will help pull out biotoxins.

Zymessence – These enzymes are incredible with inflammation and scar tissues.

Hyaluronic acid with BioCell Collagen and Collagen type 2. There are many products that are private/white labeled that have this blend. It is amazing for soft tissue damage and any injuries. It is a must have.

Dr. Schultz Intestinal formula #2 and intestinal cleanses. His incurable's program is amazing as well. Make sure to also work with cleaning and detoxing the liver. The liver has been taxed from all these toxins, bile, and the lymphatic system. Consider doing his Incurables program.

Buy iodine to help your thyroid produce all the hormones and to increase your energy.

Juice green vegetables and eliminate sugar, alcohol and gluten and also eat a healthy, mold-free diet.

Dr. Christopher's Glandular system is great if you're like me and are having trouble with your lymphatic system. This is great to rub on your neck, and it will help the sinus, tonsils and glands flush. Keep in mind you can always buy a rebounder and alternate hot and cold in the shower, always ending on cold.

Glyconutrients from Mannatech. Glyconutrients can be found in several products they offer – Ambrotose, Advanced Ambrotose and Nutriverus round out the top options. Remember these are the key nutrients that make up cell surface receptors so your body can recognize the good guys and bad guys as well as express DNA and control inflammation.

Do your own research on the things I've done and read the science for yourself online if you'd like on any of the things I've done or continue to do.

Josh Ryan

Please leave a review of this book on amazon.com so we can help more people. Remember, there are other people just like you and I that are fighting a battle from toxic mold. I put this information together to accelerate healing and wellness.

One must choose a wellness path for success in all areas of life.

ABOUT THE AUTHOR

Josh Ryan has a passion for helping and connecting with others. He's spent years doing his own study and research. He's met top Doctors and Scientists from all over the World. He believes God has provided all of the answers in nature and it's your job to act now with faith and positive expectancy. He says "no matter how long the journey, fight, winding roads or obstacles, keep faith and take massive action, what do you have to lose?"

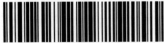

Made in the USA
Lexington, KY
02 April 2018